GLORIOUSTINA ESSIA

NATURE'S DEFENDERS

HERBAL ANTIBIOTICS AND ANTIVIRALS

This book was professionally typeset on Reedsy.
Find out more at reedsy.com

Contents

INTRODUCTION

The Rising Importance of Herbal Antibiotics and Antivirals in Modern Healthcare

In an age where the limitations of synthetic antibiotics and the rise of drug-resistant pathogens have become increasingly apparent, the quest for alternative treatments has led to a resurgence of interest in herbal medicine. "Nature's Defenders: Herbal Antibiotics and Antivirals" marks a crucial point in this journey, delving into the rich world of plant-based remedies that have stood the test of time. This book highlights the growing importance of these natural remedies in modern healthcare, offering a compelling alternative to conventional treatments.

The alarming rate at which bacteria develop antibiotic resistance is a global health concern. The overprescription and misuse of antibiotics have accelerated this process, leading to situations where common infections become deadly due to the lack of effective treatments. In this dire context, herbal antibiotics emerge as a complementary approach and a potential solution to fill gaps that modern medicine currently faces.

Similarly, the quest for antiviral treatments has been fraught with challenges. Viral diseases, ranging from the common flu to more severe conditions like HIV/AIDS and COVID-19, have shown the limits of pharmaceutical interventions. Herbal antivirals offer a spectrum of benefits, often with fewer side effects, and provide an additional arsenal in the fight against viral infections.

Historically, cultures have relied on herbal medicines to treat infections and diseases. These traditional practices, refined over centuries, are now being revisited and validated by scientific research. Compounds found in plants such as echinacea, garlic, elderberry, and turmeric have demonstrated significant antimicrobial and antiviral properties, offering a natural means to enhance the body's ability to fight infections.

The scope of "Nature's Defenders" extends beyond just listing herbal alternatives; it seeks to understand the science behind how these plants work. It dives into the phytochemical makeup of herbs, their modes of action, and the synergy of their compounds. This scientific approach legitimises herbal medicine as more than just folklore or alternative therapy but an integral part of holistic healthcare.

Moreover, this book addresses the safe and effective use of herbal antibiotics and antivirals. Understanding dosages, preparation methods, and potential interactions with conventional medications is vital for healthcare professionals and individuals seeking to incorporate these remedies into their health regimen.

CHAPTER 1: UNDERSTANDING HERBAL ANTIBIOTICS

The Science Behind Natural Antibacterial Agents

In the realm of herbal medicine, antibiotics occupy a critical place. Far from being a modern invention, using plants to combat bacterial infections has a long history, rooted in traditional medicine systems worldwide. This chapter delves into the science behind herbal antibiotics, exploring their mechanisms, efficacy, and potential in contemporary healthcare.

The Mechanism of Herbal Antibiotics

Herbal antibiotics work differently from synthetic antibiotics. While synthetic antibiotics typically target specific bacterial structures or processes, herbal antibiotics often have a broader spectrum of action. They contain compounds that can act synergistically to inhibit bacterial growth and proliferation. These natural compounds, such as alkaloids, tannins, flavonoids, and essential oils, can interfere with bacterial cell walls, disrupt protein synthesis, or inhibit specific enzymes essential for bacterial survival.

Phytochemicals in Action

The effectiveness of herbal antibiotics can be attributed to their rich phytochemical content. For instance, allicin, found in garlic, is known for its potent antibacterial properties, effective against various bacteria, including drug-resistant strains. Berberine, present in herbs like goldenseal, barberry, and Oregon grape, has been shown to combat bacteria by inhibiting their ability to adhere to human cells.

The Role of Synergy

One of the unique aspects of herbal antibiotics is the synergy of their constituent compounds. Unlike synthetic antibiotics that usually contain a single active ingredient, herbal remedies have multiple components that enhance the therapeutic effect. This synergy can make herbal antibiotics effective against a broad range of bacteria and reduce the risk of resistance development.

Research and Studies

Recent scientific research has begun to validate the efficacy of many traditional herbal remedies. Studies have shown that herbs like echinacea, thyme, and clove exhibit significant antibacterial activity. Researchers are exploring the potential of these herbs not only as standalone treatments but also as complementary therapies to enhance the effectiveness of conventional antibiotics.

Safety and Resistance

A significant advantage of herbal antibiotics is their relative safety compared to synthetic antibiotics. They are less likely to disrupt the body's natural microbiome and are generally well-tolerated. Moreover, the complex nature of herbal medicines makes it harder for bacteria to develop resistance, a major concern with synthetic antibiotics.

Challenges and Future Directions

Despite their potential, the use of herbal antibiotics is not without challenges. Standardizing dosages, quality control, and clinical trials to establish efficacy and safety require further development.

Hence, understanding herbal antibiotics is about recognizing the immense potential of nature's pharmacy. As modern medicine grapples with the challenges of antibiotic resistance, the science behind natural antibacterial agents provides a hopeful avenue for sustainable and effective solutions.

CHAPTER 2: EXPLORING HERBAL ANTIVIRALS

Mechanisms and Effectiveness in Disease Prevention

In the ongoing battle against viral diseases, herbal antivirals present a promising frontier. Unlike their pharmaceutical counterparts, these plant-based remedies offer a holistic approach, often with fewer side effects.

Understanding Viral Infections

To appreciate the role of herbal antivirals, it's crucial to understand how viral infections occur. Viruses are tiny infectious agents that invade and replicate within host cells. They can cause a range of illnesses, from the common cold and flu to more severe diseases like HIV and COVID-19. The body's natural defence against these viral invaders is the immune system, which herbal antivirals can support and enhance.

Mechanisms of Herbal Antivirals

Herbal antivirals operate through various mechanisms. Some may inhibit the ability of viruses to attach to and enter host cells. Others might interfere with viral replication or strengthen the body's immune response. For example, elderberry is known for its effectiveness against the flu virus. It prevents the virus from entering cells and boosts the production of cytokines, key immune system messengers.

Key Herbal Antivirals

Numerous herbs have been studied for their antiviral properties. Elderberry, echinacea, and astragalus are among the most well-known. Licorice root contains glycyrrhizin, which has shown effectiveness against viruses like SARS and HIV. St. John's Wort, typically known for its antidepressant properties, also contains hypericin, which may have antiviral activities against certain enveloped viruses.

Efficacy in Disease Prevention

The efficacy of herbal antivirals in disease prevention has been a subject of significant interest. Many studies have shown positive results, such as reduced duration and severity of symptoms in viral illnesses like the flu. However, it's important to note that while these herbs can be effective, they are not a substitute for vaccination or conventional medical treatment for severe viral infections.

Integrating Herbal Antivirals into Daily Life

Incorporating herbal antivirals into daily life can be a proactive measure in enhancing the body's resistance to viral infections. This can be through dietary supplements, herbal teas, or incorporating these herbs into daily meals. Understanding the appropriate dosages and considering any potential interactions with other medications is important.

CHAPTER 3: TOP HERBAL ANTIBIOTICS

Profiles and Applications of Potent Herbal Antibacterials

The world of natural medicine is abundant with plants possessing potent antibacterial properties. These herbal antibiotics have been used for centuries across various cultures to combat infections.

1. Garlic (Allium sativum)

- **Profile:** Garlic, a staple in kitchens worldwide, is renowned for its potent antibacterial properties, primarily attributed to a compound called allicin.
- **Applications:** Garlic is effective against many bacteria, including antibiotic-resistant strains. It can be used in its raw form, as a supplement, or as an oil. It's particularly useful for respiratory and gastrointestinal infections.

2. Echinacea (Echinacea spp.)

- **Profile:** Echinacea, a native North American plant, is well-known for its ability to boost the immune system and fight bacterial infections, especially in the respiratory tract.
- **Applications:** Echinacea is often used to prevent or treat colds and flu. It can be taken as a tea, tincture, or capsule. It's most effective when used at

the onset of symptoms.

3. Goldenseal (Hydrastis canadensis)

- **Profile:** Goldenseal contains berberine, a compound with strong antibacterial and anti-inflammatory properties.
- **Applications:** It is particularly effective in treating infections of the mucous membranes, including respiratory and digestive tract infections. Goldenseal is available as a tincture, capsule, or cream.

4. Thyme (Thymus vulgaris)

- **Profile:** Thyme contains thymol and carvacrol, compounds with significant antibacterial activity.
- **Applications:** Thyme is effective against respiratory infections and is often used in mouthwashes and throat lozenges. Thyme oil can be diluted and applied topically for skin infections.

5. Oregano (Origanum vulgare)

- **Profile:** Oregano, particularly its oil, is rich in carvacrol and thymol, which have broad-spectrum antibacterial properties.
- **Applications:** Oregano oil can treat gastrointestinal, respiratory, and skin infections. It is potent and should be diluted before use.

6. Honey, especially Manuka Honey

- **Profile:** Manuka honey, native to New Zealand, possesses unique antibacterial properties, making it more effective than regular honey in treating infections.
- **Applications:** Applied topically, it can treat wounds, burns, and skin infections. Ingested, it can soothe sore throats and digestive issues.

7. Ginger (Zingiber officinale)

- **Profile:** Ginger's antibacterial properties are attributed to compounds like gingerol. It is particularly effective against gastrointestinal bacteria.
- **Applications:** Ginger can be consumed fresh, as a tea, or in extract form to combat gastrointestinal infections and boost overall immunity.

8. Turmeric (Curcuma longa)

- **Profile:** The active compound in turmeric, curcumin, has potent antibacterial and anti-inflammatory properties.
- **Applications:** It's beneficial for digestive and respiratory infections and can be used in cooking, as a supplement, or applied topically in a paste.

These herbal antibiotics offer a natural alternative to synthetic antibiotics and can be a valuable part of one's health regimen. However, it is important to use them wisely and consult healthcare professionals, especially in cases of severe infection or if used in conjunction with other medications.

CHAPTER 4: HERBAL ANTIVIRALS AND THEIR HEALING PROPERTIES

In a world where viral infections are a major health concern, the importance of antiviral herbs cannot be overstated. Herbal antivirals offer a natural way to bolster the body's defences against viruses. This chapter provides a comprehensive overview of notable antiviral herbs, detailing their healing properties and how they can be incorporated into health regimens.

1. Elderberry (Sambucus nigra)

- **Profile:** Elderberry is celebrated for its antiviral properties, particularly against the flu virus. It contains compounds inhibiting virus entry and replication in human cells.
- **Uses:** Elderberry is commonly taken as a syrup or tea and is especially effective when used at the onset of flu symptoms.

2. Echinacea (Echinacea spp.)

- **Profile:** Known for boosting the immune system, Echinacea has effectively reduced the duration and severity of cold and flu symptoms.
- **Uses:** Available as capsules, tinctures, or teas, it's most beneficial when taken at the first sign of a cold.

3. Licorice Root (Glycyrrhiza glabra)

- **Profile:** Licorice root contains glycyrrhizin, which has shown antiviral activity against viruses like SARS and hepatitis.
- **Uses:** It can be consumed as a tea or in extract form but should be used cautiously due to potential side effects at high doses.

4. St. John's Wort (Hypericum perforatum)

- **Profile:** Beyond its antidepressant properties, St. John's Wort has components that exhibit antiviral activity, particularly against enveloped viruses.
- **Uses:** Commonly taken as capsules or tinctures, it's crucial to note its interactions with various medications.

5. Astragalus (Astragalus membranaceus)

- **Profile:** Astragalus is a staple in traditional Chinese medicine, known for its immune-boosting and antiviral properties.
- **Uses:** It can be added to soups, as a supplement, or as a tincture, particularly during cold and flu season.

6. Garlic (Allium sativum)

- **Profile:** Garlic has broad-spectrum antimicrobial and antiviral properties. It's particularly effective against respiratory infections.
- **Uses:** Consuming raw garlic, garlic capsules, or aged garlic extract can help fend off viral infections.

7. Lemon Balm (Melissa officinalis)

- **Profile:** Lemon balm has antiviral effects against herpes simplex virus and other viruses.
- **Uses:** It can be applied topically in cream form for herpes outbreaks or consumed as tea for its calming effects.

8. Oregano (Origanum vulgare) and Oregano Oil

- **Profile:** Oregano and its oil are rich in compounds like carvacrol, which exhibit antiviral properties.
- **Uses:** Oregano oil is potent and should be diluted if used topically or orally for respiratory infections.

Using herbal antivirals is an age-old practice that remains relevant in modern times. Each of these herbs offers unique antiviral properties and can be a valuable addition to one's health arsenal, especially in preventing and mitigating viral infections. While these herbs are generally safe, it is crucial to use them judiciously, respecting their potency and potential interactions with other medications.

CHAPTER 5: LESSER-KNOWN HERBAL ANTIBIOTICS AND ANTIVIRALS

Exploring Underutilized but Effective Remedies

While some herbal remedies like garlic and echinacea are widely recognized for their antibacterial and antiviral properties, numerous lesser-known herbs are equally potent but remain underutilized. This chapter sheds light on these hidden gems of the herbal world, exploring their unique properties and how they can contribute to health and wellness.

1. Andrographis (Andrographis paniculata)

- **Profile:** Often referred to as 'Indian Echinacea,' Andrographis is a potent herb used traditionally in Ayurvedic and Chinese medicine. It's known for its strong antibacterial and antiviral properties, particularly effective in treating respiratory infections like colds and flu.
- **Uses:** Typically consumed in capsule or extract form, it's best taken at the onset of symptoms.

2. Olive Leaf (Olea europaea)

- **Profile:** The leaf of the olive tree contains oleuropein, a compound with significant antimicrobial and antiviral activities. It's particularly effective against respiratory infections and has been studied for its potential in treating viral illnesses.
- **Uses:** Olive leaf can be consumed as a tea, extract, or capsule form.

3. Pau D'Arco (Tabebuia impetiginosa)

- **Profile:** This South American herb has potent antifungal and antiviral properties. It contains naphthoquinones, compounds that can inhibit the growth of viruses and bacteria.
- **Uses:** Pau D'Arco is typically consumed as a tea or extract and is often used to treat candida overgrowths and other fungal infections.

4. Usnea (Usnea spp.)

- **Profile:** Also known as Old Man's Beard, Usnea is a lichen that grows on trees and possesses potent antibacterial and antiviral properties, particularly against respiratory and skin infections.
- **Uses:** It's usually prepared as a tincture and used topically and internally.

5. Baikal Skullcap (Scutellaria baicalensis)

- **Profile:** A staple in traditional Chinese medicine, Baikal skullcap has compounds like baicalin that exhibit strong antibacterial and antiviral effects, especially against respiratory infections.
- **Uses:** It's commonly consumed as a tea or extract.

6. Neem (Azadirachta indica)

- **Profile:** Neem, a cornerstone in Ayurvedic medicine, has broad-spectrum antimicrobial properties. It's particularly noted for its antiviral activity against smallpox and chickenpox viruses.
- **Uses:** Neem leaves can be consumed as a tea or used topically as an oil for skin infections.

7. Cat's Claw (Uncaria tomentosa)

- **Profile:** This vine from the Amazon rainforest is known for boosting the immune system and fighting off viral infections, including herpes and HIV.
- **Uses:** Cat's Claw is usually taken in capsule form or as a tea.

8. Rhodiola (Rhodiola rosea)

- **Profile:** Known primarily for its adaptogenic properties, Rhodiola also has antiviral capabilities, particularly in combating fatigue associated with viral infections.
- **Uses:** It's typically taken as a supplement or extract.

These lesser-known herbs represent just a fraction of the vast potential that natural medicine holds. Incorporating these underutilized herbs into health practices can provide effective alternatives or complements to conventional antibiotics and antivirals. However, it's important to approach their use with knowledge and caution, ideally under the guidance of a healthcare professional, especially for individuals with existing health conditions or those taking other medications.

CHAPTER 6: DIY RECIPES AND EXTRACTION METHODS

Harnessing the power of herbal antibiotics and antivirals requires more than just knowledge of their benefits; it also involves understanding how to prepare them effectively.

1. Decoctions and Infusions

- **Basics:** Decoctions and infusions are simple yet effective ways to extract the medicinal properties of herbs. Decoctions are made by boiling tougher plant parts like roots and bark, whereas infusions are akin to teas, steeping the more delicate parts like leaves and flowers in hot water.
- **Recipe:** For a basic decoction, simmer one dried herb in ten parts of water until the volume is reduced by half. For an infusion, steep one teaspoon of dried herb in one cup of hot water for 10–15 minutes.

2. Tinctures

- **Overview:** Tinctures are concentrated herbal extracts made using alcohol or glycerin. They offer a longer shelf life and can be more potent than teas.
- **DIY Method:** Combine one dried herb with four parts alcohol (like vodka or brandy) or glycerin. Store in a dark glass jar, shake daily, and strain after 4-6 weeks.

3. Herbal Syrups

- **Benefits:** Syrups are a pleasant way to take herbal remedies, especially suitable for children or those opposed to the taste of tinctures.
- **Recipe:** Make a strong decoction, then add equal parts honey or sugar. Gently heat until the sweetener dissolves. Bottle and refrigerate.

4. Herbal Oils and Salves

- **Usefulness:** For topical application, herbal oils and salves are ideal for skin infections and irritations.
- **Preparation:** Infuse herbs in a carrier oil (like olive or coconut oil) in a double boiler for 2–3 hours. Strain and store. Add beeswax to the strained oil and pour into containers to solidify for salves.

5. Herbal Capsules

- **Convenience:** Capsules offer a convenient way to consume herbal antibiotics and antivirals, especially for those with a busy lifestyle.
- **Method:** Powder-dried herbs using a grinder. Use a capsule machine to fill empty capsules with the powder.

6. Herbal Steam Inhalations

- **For Respiratory Issues:** Steam inhalations are effective for respiratory infections.
- **Technique:** Boil water with herbs like eucalyptus or thyme. Remove from heat, cover your head with a towel, and inhale the steam.

7. Herbal Gargles and Mouthwashes

- **Oral Health:** Useful for sore throats and oral infections.
- **Recipe:** Make a strong infusion with antibacterial herbs like sage or calendula. Cool, strain, and use as a gargle or mouthwash.

Preparing herbal antibiotics and antivirals can be a fulfilling and effective way to manage health naturally. These DIY methods not only provide a hands-on approach to herbal medicine but also allow customization according to individual needs and preferences. While preparing these remedies, it's essential to source high-quality herbs and adhere to safety guidelines, ensuring the most beneficial and potent results from your herbal preparations.

CHAPTER 7: GUIDELINES FOR SAFE AND EFFECTIVE USE

Navigating the world of herbal antibiotics and antivirals involves more than just understanding their benefits; it's also crucial to know about proper Dosage, administration, and safety.

1. Understanding Dosage

- **Importance of Correct Dosage:** The efficacy of an herbal remedy is significantly influenced by its Dosage. Too little may be ineffective, while too much could lead to adverse effects.
- **Factors to Consider:** Dosage depends on age, weight, health condition, and the herb's potency. It's often best to start with a lower dose and gradually increase as needed.

2. Methods of Administration

- **Various Forms:** Herbal remedies can be administered in several forms, including teas, tinctures, capsules, oils, and topicals. The choice depends on the condition being treated and personal preference.
- **Duration of Use:** Some herbs are suitable for long-term use, while others should be used only for short periods. It's important to research or consult a professional about the recommended duration for each herb.

3. Safety Considerations

- **Side Effects:** While herbal remedies are generally safe, they can cause side effects or allergic reactions in some individuals. Awareness of common side effects associated with specific herbs is important.
- **Interactions with Medications:** Some herbs can interact with prescription medications, either enhancing or inhibiting their effects. Always consult a healthcare provider before combining herbal remedies with prescription drugs.

4. Special Populations

- **Pregnancy and Breastfeeding:** Caution is advised when using herbal remedies during pregnancy and breastfeeding. Some herbs can be harmful to the developing fetus or nursing infant.
- **Children and the Elderly:** Dosages for children and the elderly should be adjusted, as their bodies process substances differently. Professional guidance is recommended.

5. Quality of Herbs

- **Source Responsibly:** The quality of herbal remedies is crucial for their efficacy and safety. Source herbs from reputable suppliers to ensure they are free from contaminants and pollutants.
- **Organic and Wildcrafted:** Choose organic or responsibly wildcrafted herbs to minimize exposure to pesticides and environmental toxins whenever possible.

6. Storage and Shelf Life

- **Proper Storage:** Herbs and preparations should be stored properly to maintain potency. Most dried herbs and capsules should be kept in a cool, dark place, while tinctures and oils may have different storage requirements.

- **Shelf Life Awareness:** Be aware of the shelf life of different herbal preparations. While dried herbs can last up to two years, preparations like tinctures and oils may have longer or shorter shelf lives.

Responsible use of herbal antibiotics and antivirals is key to maximizing their benefits while minimizing risks. By understanding and adhering to guidelines on Dosage, administration, and safety, individuals can confidently incorporate these natural remedies into their health regimen. When in doubt, consult with a healthcare professional, especially for serious health conditions, to ensure the effective use of herbal remedies.

CHAPTER 8: CREATING A HERBAL FIRST-AID KIT

Essentials for Home and Travel

An herbal first-aid kit is invaluable for naturally addressing minor ailments at home and while travelling. This chapter guides you through assembling a versatile and effective herbal first-aid kit, ensuring you're prepared for common health issues with natural remedies.

1. Selecting a Container

- **Compact and Portable:** Choose a container that is both sturdy and portable. A small backpack, a box with compartments, or a pouch are all suitable options, depending on your space and mode of travel.

2. Essential Herbal Remedies

- **For Cuts and Wounds:** Include antiseptic herbs like calendula and yarrow, which can be used as salves or tinctures. These herbs aid in wound healing and prevent infection.
- **Digestive Aids:** Ginger capsules or tea for nausea, chamomile tea for stomach upset, and activated charcoal for food poisoning.
- **Respiratory Relief:** Eucalyptus oil for decongestion, elderberry syrup for

colds and flu, and peppermint tea for sore throats.

- **Pain and Inflammation:** Arnica cream for bruises and sore muscles, white willow bark capsules as a natural pain reliever, and turmeric capsules for anti-inflammatory needs.
- **Skin Irritations:** Aloe vera gel for burns and sunburn, tea tree oil for antifungal needs, and lavender essential oil for bug bites and stings.
- **Sleep and Relaxation:** Valerian root capsules or lemon balm tea for insomnia and stress relief.

3. Herbal First-Aid Accessories

- **Bandages and Gauze:** For covering and protecting wounds.
- **Cotton Swabs and Balls:** For applying herbal tinctures and oils.
- **Tweezers and Scissors:** For removing splinters and cutting bandages.
- **A Small Notebook:** Containing information on the use and dosage of each herb and remedy in your kit.

4. Customizing Your Kit

- **Personal Needs:** Tailor your kit to address personal or family-specific health needs. If you frequently encounter allergies, include nettle capsules or quercetin.
- **Local Flora:** If travelling, research the local flora and potential herbal remedies specific to that region.

5. Safe Storage and Shelf Life

- **Proper Storage:** Keep your kit in a cool, dry place to preserve the potency of the herbs. Avoid leaving it in direct sunlight or a hot vehicle.
- **Shelf Life Awareness:** Regularly check and replace items past their expiration date or lost potency.

6. Educating Yourself and Others

- **Knowledge is Key:** Familiarize yourself with the uses and dosages of the items in your kit. Consider including a small guide or notes for quick reference.
- **Training:** Basic knowledge of first aid is beneficial. Knowing when to use your herbal remedies and when to seek medical attention is crucial.

A well-prepared herbal first-aid kit is a practical and empowering tool for addressing everyday health concerns. It ensures you have natural, effective remedies at home or on the go. Remember, while herbal remedies are excellent for minor ailments, they are not substitutes for professional medical care in emergencies.

CHAPTER 9: INCORPORATING HERBS INTO DAILY LIFE

Integrating Herbal Antibiotics into Health Regimens

Incorporating herbal antibiotics into daily health routines effectively enhances immune function and guards against infections. This chapter focuses on seamlessly integrating these natural remedies into your everyday life, ensuring a holistic approach to wellness.

1. Understanding Herbal Antibiotics

- **Basics of Herbal Antibiotics:** Herbal antibiotics are natural substances derived from plants with antimicrobial properties. Unlike pharmaceutical antibiotics, they often strengthen the body's immune system and create an environment less favourable for bacterial growth.
- **Active Constituents:** Familiarize yourself with the active constituents in herbal antibiotics, such as allicin in garlic or berberine in goldenseal, and their specific effects on the body.

2. Daily Integration Strategies

- **Dietary Incorporation:** One of the easiest ways to include herbal antibiotics in your regimen is through your diet. Add garlic, onions, ginger, and turmeric to your meals for their antimicrobial benefits.
- **Herbal Teas:** Regularly consuming herbal teas like echinacea, elderberry, and green tea can provide immune support.
- **Tinctures and Supplements:** Consider herbal tinctures or supplements for more potent effects. These concentrated forms can be preventive measures during cold and flu season.

3. Preventive vs. Reactive Use

- **Preventive Use:** Regular, low-dose intake of certain herbal antibiotics can help maintain a robust immune system. For instance, astragalus is known for its ability to enhance immune function when used preventively.
- **Reactive Use:** Increase the use of specific herbs at the first sign of an infection. For example, high doses of echinacea can be effective at the onset of a cold.

4. Synergistic Combinations

- **Combining Herbs:** Some herbs work better in combination. For instance, combining echinacea with goldenseal can enhance the immune-boosting effect.
- **Whole-Body Support:** Consider herbs that support other systems, like the digestive or respiratory system, for overall health.

5. Lifestyle Considerations

- **Stress Management:** Chronic stress can weaken the immune system. Integrating adaptogenic herbs like ashwagandha or Rhodiola can help the body cope with stress.

- **Physical Activity:** Regular exercise can boost your immune system. Pairing physical activity with a diet rich in herbal antibiotics creates a strong defence against infections.

6. Safety and Consultation

- **Professional Advice:** Always consult with a healthcare provider, especially if you have existing health conditions or are on medication. Some herbal antibiotics can interact with pharmaceuticals.
- **Allergies and Side Effects:** Be aware of potential allergies or side effects. Start with small doses to test your body's reaction.

7. Educating Yourself

- **Stay Informed:** Continuously educate yourself about herbal medicine. Read reputable books, attend workshops, or consult with herbalists to deepen your understanding.

Integrating herbal antibiotics into your health regimen is a proactive step towards enhanced well-being. Incorporating these natural defenders into your daily routine supports your immune system's ability to ward off infections and maintain overall health. Remember, the key to effective use lies in understanding, consistency, and balance, ensuring that these natural remedies complement a healthy lifestyle.

CHAPTER 10: BALANCED APPROACH TO HEALTH AND WELLNESS

In the pursuit of optimal health, combining herbal and conventional treatments offers a holistic approach. This chapter explores how to synergistically use both modalities, striking a balance that maximizes the benefits of each system while minimizing potential risks.

1. The Integrative Health Perspective

- **Philosophy of Integration:** Integrative health combines the best of conventional medicine and alternative therapies, including herbal remedies. This approach focuses on treating the whole person - body, mind, and spirit.
- **Personalized Treatment:** Every individual's health needs are unique. Integrative health tailors treatments, combining the precision of conventional medicine with the holistic benefits of herbal remedies.

2. Understanding Interactions

- **Herb-Drug Interactions:** One of the key concerns in combining treatments is the potential for interactions. Certain herbs can amplify or diminish the effects of pharmaceutical drugs.
- **Informed Decisions:** Stay informed about how specific herbs interact with medications. For example, St. John's Wort can interfere with the

effectiveness of certain antidepressants and birth control pills.

3. Coordinated Health Care

- **Communicate with Health Care Providers:** Transparency with healthcare providers is crucial. Inform doctors and herbalists about all the treatments you are using.
- **Collaborative Care:** Seek healthcare professionals open to an integrative approach and can help coordinate your care between different modalities.

4. Complementing Conventional Treatments with Herbs

- **Supportive Role of Herbs:** Use herbal remedies to support conventional treatments. For instance, ginger can be used to alleviate nausea associated with chemotherapy.
- **Enhancing Well-being:** Herbs can enhance overall well-being, such as using adaptogenic herbs to reduce stress or improve sleep quality.

5. Safely Navigating Herbal Treatments

- **Quality and Purity:** Ensure herbal products are from reputable sources to guarantee purity and potency.
- **Start Low and Go Slow:** When introducing new herbal remedies, start with lower doses and gradually increase, monitoring for adverse reactions or interactions.

6. The Role of Preventive Care

- **Preventive Approach:** Herbal remedies can be used proactively to strengthen the body's natural defences, potentially reducing the need for conventional medications.
- **Lifestyle Integration:** Combine herbal treatments with healthy lifestyle choices, such as a balanced diet, regular exercise, and stress management

techniques.

7. Addressing Chronic Conditions

- **Managing Chronic Illness:** In cases of chronic illness, herbs can be used to manage symptoms and improve quality of life, complementing conventional care.
- **Continuous Monitoring:** Regular monitoring and adjustments by health-care professionals are essential to ensure the effectiveness and safety of combined treatments.

CHAPTER 11: BUILDING NATURAL IMMUNITY WITH HERBS

Long-Term Strategies for Health and Disease Prevention

The role of herbs in enhancing and maintaining a robust immune system cannot be overstated. Utilizing herbs as a long-term health and disease prevention strategy is wise and practical in a world of ever-evolving health challenges.

1. Understanding Immune Function

- **Immune System Basics:** The immune system is a complex network of cells, tissues, and organs that work together to defend the body against pathogens.
- **Herbs and Immunity:** Certain herbs possess properties that can support and modulate immune function, making the body more efficient at combating infections and diseases.

2. Key Immune-Boosting Herbs

- **Astragalus (Astragalus membranaceus):** Known for its immune-enhancing properties, astragalus is used to prevent colds and respiratory infections.

- **Echinacea (Echinacea spp.):** Popular for its ability to fight the common cold and flu, echinacea can improve immune health when used regularly.
- **Ginseng (Panax ginseng):** Renowned for boosting energy and immune function, ginseng is a valuable herb for overall vitality.
- **Elderberry (Sambucus nigra):** Elderberry's antiviral properties make it effective in preventing and easing flu symptoms.
- **Garlic (Allium sativum):** With potent antimicrobial properties, garlic is a powerhouse for immune support.

3. Incorporating Herbs into Daily Regimens

- **Dietary Integration:** Add immune-boosting herbs to your diet through cooking, teas, and supplements.
- **Herbal Supplements:** For more concentrated benefits, herbal supplements can be convenient. Ensure they are sourced from reputable suppliers.
- **Seasonal Use:** Some herbs are particularly beneficial when used in specific seasons. For instance, echinacea during flu season.

4. Supporting Overall Health

- **Holistic Approach:** Immune health is tied to overall well-being. Support your immune system by maintaining a healthy diet, exercising regularly, and managing stress.
- **Gut Health:** As a significant portion of the immune system resides in the gut, herbs that support digestive health can also benefit immunity.

5. Long-Term Use and Cycles

- **Sustainable Use:** Some immune-boosting herbs are best used in cycles or for limited periods to maintain effectiveness and prevent immune system overstimulation.
- **Adaptogens:** Herbs like ashwagandha and Rhodiola help the body adapt

to stress and can be used long-term for sustained immune support.

6. Safety and Interactions

- **Consult Healthcare Providers:** Always consult with a healthcare professional before starting any new herbal regimen, especially if you have existing health conditions or are taking medications.
- **Awareness of Side Effects:** Be aware of potential side effects and allergic reactions. Start with small doses to test tolerance.

7. Customizing Herbal Strategies

- **Personal Needs:** Tailor your herbal regimen to suit your health needs, lifestyle, and preferences. What works for one person might not work for another.

CONCLUSION

This book has illuminated herbs' potent capabilities in combating infections and reinforced the importance of integrating these ancient remedies into modern health practices.

In these pages, we've journeyed across cultures and centuries, unravelling the secrets of herbs that have defended human health long before the advent of synthetic medicines. From the immune-boosting echinacea to the antiviral prowess of elderberry, the natural world offers a pharmacy of its own, rich in remedies waiting to be rediscovered and embraced.

This exploration is more than a compilation of herbal facts and recipes; it is a call to reconnect with nature's wisdom, to blend tradition with science, and to foster a deeper understanding of how nature's bounty can be harnessed for better health. "Nature's Defenders" encourages a proactive approach to wellness, emphasizing the role of herbal antibiotics and antivirals as allies in an era where the resilience of our immune systems has never been more crucial.

As readers, you are equipped with knowledge and the tools to make informed decisions about your health and well-being. Whether incorporating garlic into your diet for its antimicrobial properties, brewing a cup of ginger tea to ward off a cold, or turning to astragalus for immune support, your everyday choices can shape your health journey.

In a world where health is a balance of mind, body, and spirit, "Nature's Defenders" serves as a testament to the power of herbal medicine, a bridge between the ancient and the modern, and a guide for those seeking a more holistic, natural path to wellness. May this book inspire you to explore herbs' healing powers and embrace them as a part of a balanced, healthful life.

Remember, the journey with herbal medicine is continuous, one of learning, experiencing, and growing.

SOURCES

https://www.healthline.com/health/natural-antibiotics#takeaway

https://study.com/academy/lesson/what-is-a-natural-antibiotic-foods-plants.html

https://www.ncbi.nlm.nih.gov/pmc/articles/PMC9554739/

https://pubmed.ncbi.nlm.nih.gov/35184680/

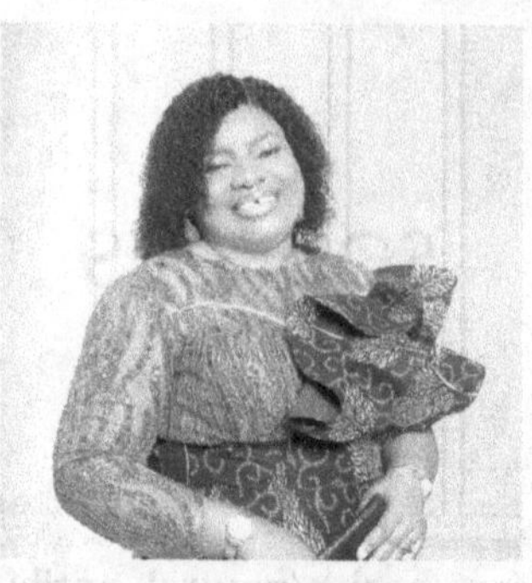

About the Author

Glorioustina Essia is a multifaceted professional whose expertise traverses the realms of technology, artificial intelligence, literature, and natural health. As a driving force in artificial intelligence, particularly in prompt engineering, she has established herself as a pioneer. Her proficiency extends to project management, network marketing, website development, and copywriting, showcasing a unique blend of technical understanding and creative flair.

A prolific author and publisher, Glorioustina's literary works span multiple genres, captivating a diverse audience with her narrative skill and inspiring a new generation of writers to unlock their creative potential. Her passion for storytelling matches her commitment to exploring and advocating for holistic health practices. Renowned in herbal medicine, she dedicates her life to studying and promoting natural health.

Glorioustina Essia's professional and personal journey is characterized by an unwavering dedication to her core strengths and a ceaseless pursuit of knowledge. Her zeal and expertise embody the limitless possibilities that arise from a commitment to innovation, quality, and a deep-seated passion for understanding the future of technology and the ancient wisdom of herbal medicine. Glorioustina is a testament to the power of interdisciplinary knowledge and its impact in a world where technology, literature, and natural health converge.

You can connect with me on:

🌐 https://www.amazon.com/author/glorioustina

Also by GLORIOUSTINA ESSIA

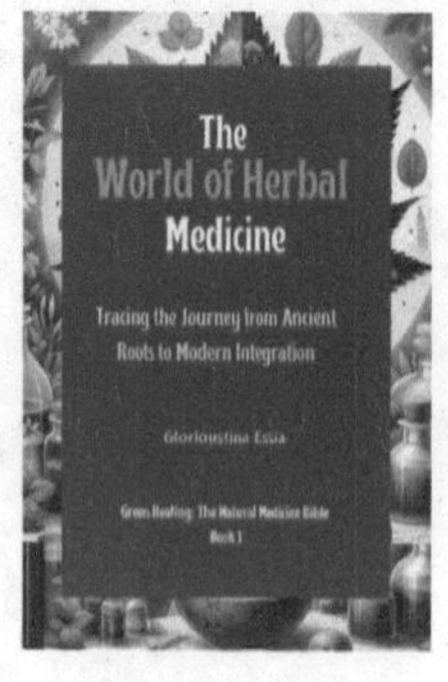

The World of Herbal Medicine

In an era where the rush of modern medicine often overshadows the pursuit of holistic health, the timeless wisdom of herbal remedies remains largely untapped. Do you find yourself seeking a more natural approach to health and wellness yet still determining where to begin or how to integrate these practices with modern healthcare?

Embark on a transformative journey with Book 1 of "Green Healing: The Natural Medicine Bible": "The World of Herbal Medicine." This enlightening volume takes you through the ancient pathways to the modern integration of herbal healing. Discover herbal medicine's rich history and evolution across different cultures, including the profound insights of Traditional Chinese Medicine, Ayurveda, and indigenous practices. Unravel how herbalism has evolved through historical epochs and how it beautifully intersects with modern medical practices today.

Embrace the journey to holistic health – add this captivating volume to your collection and begin exploring the world of herbal medicine today

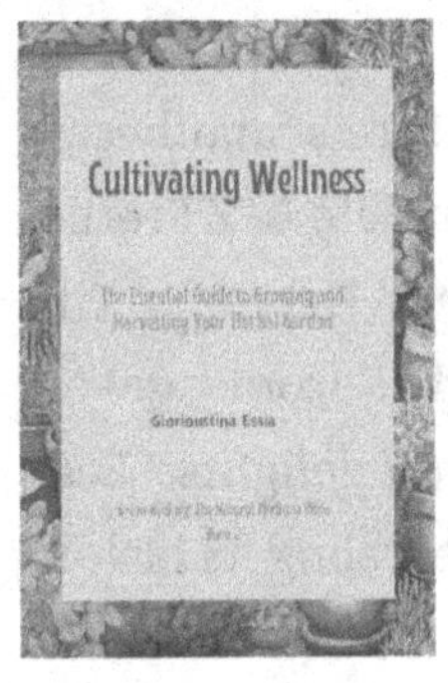

Cultivating Wellness

This guide is your gateway to mastering the art of herb gardening, offering practical advice for cultivating various medicinal and culinary herbs. From sustainable techniques to harvesting and preservation methods, each chapter brims with expert knowledge tailored to beginners and experienced gardeners. Learn to navigate common challenges in herb gardening and create specialized gardens for your health and culinary needs. Beyond gardening tips, this book inspires a deeper connection with nature and a commitment to a holistic lifestyle. Embrace the journey of nurturing not just a garden but a healthier, more harmonious way of life with "Cultivating Wellness."

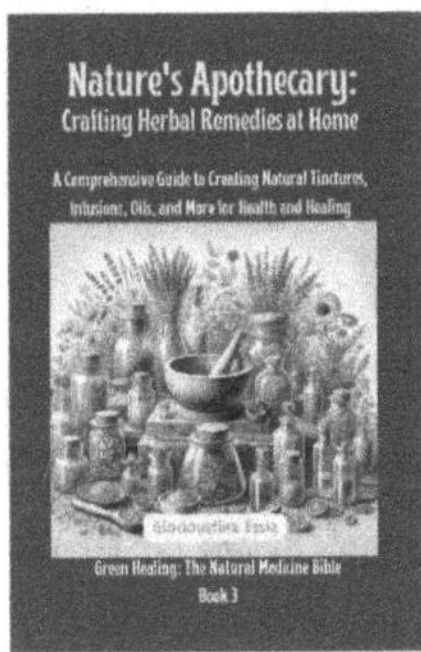

Nature's Apothecary

This comprehensive guide demystifies making your natural tinctures, infusions, oils, and more. It provides step-by-step instructions and detailed information on various herbs and their medicinal properties, empowering you to create effective, natural remedies in your kitchen.

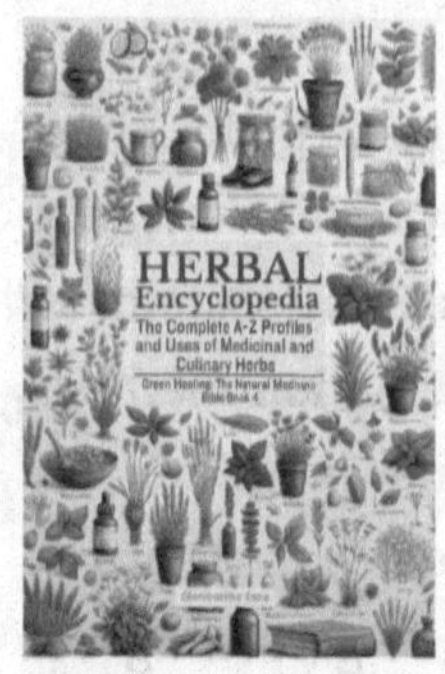

Herbal Encyclopedia

Embark on a journey through nature's apothecary with "Herbal Encyclopedia: The Complete A-Z Profiles and Uses of Medicinal and Culinary Herbs." This guide unravels the secrets of herbs, from age-old medicinal uses to enhancing culinary delights. Each page introduces you to a new herb, revealing its history, health benefits, and how it can be incorporated into your daily life. Whether you're a budding herbalist or a seasoned enthusiast, this encyclopedia offers easy-to-understand profiles, practical tips, and a connection to the ancient art of herbal healing.

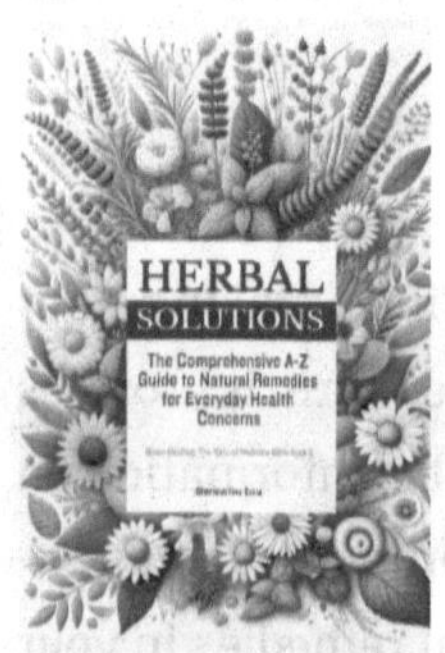

Herbal Solutions

Discover the secrets to natural wellness with "Herbal Solutions: The Comprehensive A-Z Guide to Natural Remedies for Everyday Health Concerns" This essential resource offers easy-to-access, alphabetical listings of natural remedies for a wide range of common health issues. From herbal solutions to holistic approaches, each entry provides practical, safe, and effective ways to enhance your health naturally. Perfect for those seeking alternative options or complementing traditional medicine, this guide empowers you with the knowledge to take control of your well-being.

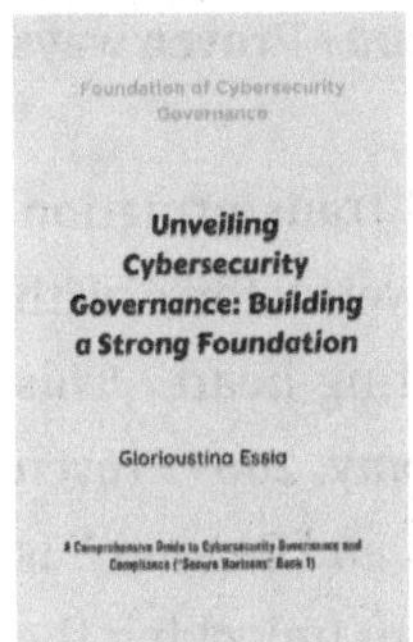

Unveiling Cybersecurity Governance

In the ever-expanding digital landscape, safeguarding sensitive information and maintaining robust cybersecurity practices have become paramount. "Unveiling Cybersecurity Governance: Building a Strong Foundation" is a comprehensive guide that delves into cybersecurity governance's core principles and components, equipping readers with the knowledge and tools to establish a secure digital environment.

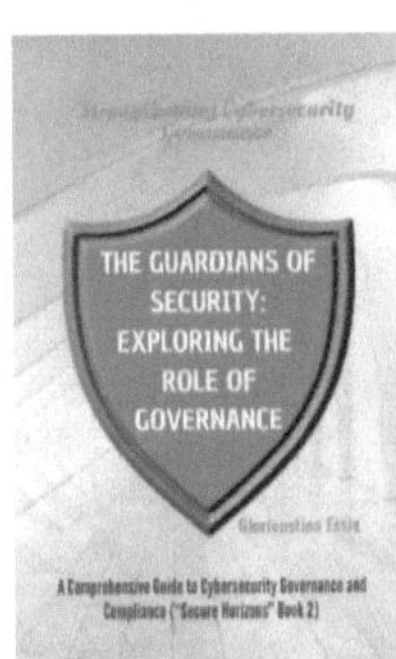

THE GUARDIANS OF SECURITY

Step into a world where cybersecurity governance catalyzes a secure future. Explore the realms of "The Guardians of Security: Exploring the Role of Governance," the much-awaited second book in the epic series "Secure Horizons: A Comprehensive Guide to Cybersecurity Governance and Compliance."

As you read each page of "The Guardians of Security," prepare to be enchanted by the author's remarkable storytelling ability. This book presents a vivid picture of the complicated landscape of cybersecurity governance with a seamless blend of real-world experiences, cutting-edge research, and visionary concepts. Immerse yourself in an exciting story that uncovers the brains and souls of people dedicated to defending our digital borders.

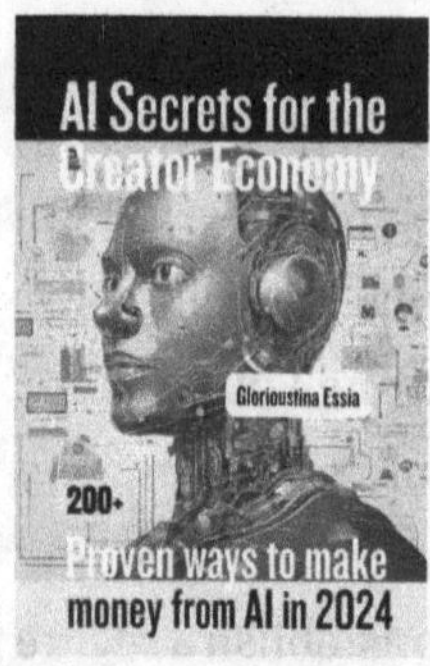

AI Secrets for the Creator Economy: 200+ Proven ways to make money from AI in 2024

In a world driven by innovation and transformation, the Creator Economy emerges as a powerful force, with Artificial Intelligence (AI) at its beating heart. This book, "AI Secrets for the Creator Economy: 200+ Proven Ways to Make Money from AI in 2024 and Beyond," is more than just a book; it's your key to unlocking the incredible synergy between AI and creativity, opening the door to a wealth of opportunities for those who are willing to seize them.

www.ingramcontent.com/pod-product-compliance
Lightning Source LLC
Chambersburg PA
CBHW012312240726
48656CB00008B/2653